john shepherd and mike antoniades

youth fitness

101

drills
age 7–11

Published in 2010 by
A & C Black Publishers Ltd
36 Soho Square
London W1D 3QY
www.acblack.com

ISBN 978 14081 1484 1

A CIP catalogue record for this book is available from the British Library.

Acknowledgements
Cover photograph © Getty Images
Textual photographs © Grant Pritchard
Illustrations by Mark Silver
Commissioning editor – Charlotte Croft
Editor – Kate Turvey
Designer – James Watson

Note
While every effort has been made to ensure that the content of this book is as technically accurate and as sound as possible, neither the authors nor the publishers can accept responsibility for any injury or loss sustained as a result of the use of this material.

A & C Black uses paper produced with elemental chlorine-free pulp, harvested from managed sustainable forests.

Typeset in 10 on 12pt Din Regular by Margaret Brain, Wisbech

Printed and bound by Martins the Printers

CONTENTS

ABOUT THE AUTHORS

John Shepherd

John Shepherd is the editor of *ultra-FIT* magazine and a freelance writer. He has written five other bestselling fitness and sports books, including *The Complete Guide to Sports Training* and *101 Youth Athletics Drills*. He is a former international athlete and coaches athletes to international standard. He still competes at master's level at sprints and long jump and has won numerous national, European and World medals.

John has also worked for local authorities in sports development, where he puts into practice many of the drills in this book.

Mike Antoniades

Mike is the founder and coaching director of Sport Dimensions and The Running School®. He is an innovative coach and an expert in speed and strength training, and rehabilitation after injury or surgery.

His reputation as a coach has seen him work with professional and elite sportspeople in football, rugby and athletics from teams such as Chelsea, Tottenham, Fulham, Blackburn, and England rugby internationals. He has worked with TV personalities and recreational athletes and has experience of working with young people in school and sports clubs.

Mike has been featured in numerous newspapers and magazines for his work with elite athletes and football clubs, such as *Running Fitness*, *The Times*, *Mirror*, *Daily Mail*, *Daily Telegraph* and *Peak Performance*. His training techniques have also been highlighted on the *BBC Sports Academy*.

He is also the author of a DVD on developing speed in football called *Feel the Speed* and runs workshops on fitness and speed development in the UK, Europe and the USA.

Putting theory into practice

Together John Shepherd and Mike Antoniades run courses designed to bring the drills and exercises in these and their other books to the attention of teachers and coaches. For further information go to: www.sportsdimensions.com

The warning signs...

More than a quarter of children in secondary schools in England are obese – that's double the number from 10 years ago. These figures, alarming as they are, become even more so when you learn that, for the National Obesity Forum*, this constitutes a 'public health time bomb' which will see obese teenagers twice as likely to die by the age of 50.

If overweight young people are added to the numbers who are obese, then a staggering 46% of girls and 30.5% of boys are overweight or obese.

We hope that *101 Youth Fitness Drills* will help to improve this alarming situation.

The recommendations

Officially the Chief Medical Officer recommends that young people aged 5-18 do at least 60 minutes of moderate activity each day. Twice a week this hour should include activities to improve muscle strength, flexibility and bone health (this would include running and jumping, dance classes and resistance exercise)**. However, the government wants all 5–18-year-olds to do four hours of quality sport/physical education a week by 2010***.

We believe that young people need two or three hours of physical activity every day! At least 60 minutes should be in bursts of high intensity – games, running, jumping. All of it should be fun. So it is up to us as parents, teachers and coaches to start educating our children and give them the tools for leading healthy, active lives.

*The National Obesity Forum was established in May 2002 to raise awareness of the growing impact of obesity and being overweight on patients and the NHS. www.nationalobesity forum.org.uk
**Donaldson L; 'At least five a week: evidence on the impact of physical activity and its relationship to health'. A report from the Chief Medical Officer. 2004, The Stationery Office
***Department of Culture, Media and Sport: www.culture.gov.uk

INTRODUCTION

Fitness should be fun, and not a chore or something you 'have to do'. This is especially true for children. Only a generation ago children played much more actively and with greater freedom. Today, concerns over health and safety at school and in the wider community, coupled with the twin malaises of the twenty-first century, poor diet and a lack of exercise, have led to huge actual and potential health concerns. Indeed the term 'globesity' has been coined to describe the problem. *101 Youth Fitness Drills* aims to help children enjoy physical activity and provide them with a foundation of skills (or what has been called 'physical literacy') so that their future will be active and health-aware.

Through our own experiences and attendance of numerous coaching courses over the years, and through talking with coaches from many sports, we know that not only are many children unhealthy, but they are also unable to perform basic physical skills that would make them better at playing sports. Turning and spinning through 180 or 360 degrees, for example, is a skill many children lack – a skill that is crucial for sports such as football and tennis, and the track and field discus throw. So another aim of this book and its sister title for the 12–16 age group is to provide an array of largely game-based drills and practices which will help a child improve whatever their sport. Hopefully – and crucially – in taking part in these drills the child will be learning in a way that does not seem like learning. We want children to have fun while they become more skilled, more body aware, faster, better coordinated and, above all, fitter.

John Shepherd   **Mike Antoniades**

CHILD DEVELOPMENT AND PHYSICAL ACTIVITY

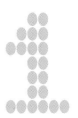

Although we have written this book to produce more confident and physically gifted children, our primary aim is to stimulate an interest in being active, regardless of whether a child wants to be a sportsperson in the future. In short, we want to encourage a healthy and active lifestyle. This is in slight contrast to the other *101 Drills* books in the series because these are aimed at giving children specific skills in, for example, rugby, netball or athletics. Although all the drills in this book will help build sports skills, they have also been selected because they are fun to do. Many are as much games as they are drills.

For many of us who are of a certain age, they will bring back memories of being scouts or guides or of our PE lessons when we played dodge ball and British bulldogs, and ran through obstacle courses. These are activities that involve a variety of valuable sports and fitness skills, but are great fun to do. It is far better to get children active and improving their physical ability without them really knowing it, than by being too formal.

your role

To make fitness fun, your role as teacher, parent or coach, is very important. You must be enthusiastic about the activities you are leading and you must be inclusive, encouraging and creative. With the 7–11 age range you'll probably find that most children are willing and able to participate in the activities. They will be much less self-aware than 12–16-year-olds, and peer pressure won't be as much of an issue. However, as the overweight and obesity figures indicate (see page v) there may well be children in your care who are less inclined to want to take part. This may be because they have not been brought up in an environment that encourages physical activity. You should keep an eye out for them and alter the way you present your session to help them feel more confident about taking part. Obviously if you have health concerns about any chldren, they should not participate or continue with the session – although we are sure this will be very rare. However, you should be aware of specific health needs, preferably before taking the session. Preventing a child from doing an activity in the heat of the moment, because of their weight, for example, could be detrimental to their self-esteem.

Nationally, special programmes have been established to work with teenagers who are overweight or obese. Find out as much as you can about what's happening in your area as you may be able to direct a child to a particular scheme – through their parent or guardian, of course.

In terms of your session or lesson you must be on the look-out for any child who is having difficulty performing the exercises and try to ensure that they are able to do them safely and to the best of their abilities.

the best times to get children fitter

There are times when children will respond to certain types of exercise better than others – this information is presented in table 1 for boys and table 2 for girls.

Why is it important to develop these physiological elements during these periods? Research shows that at these times a child's body is developing the right enzymes and hormones which will maximise the development of a particular aspect of their physiology. For example, it is argued that if not trained for speed during the appropriate windows, then a child will never be able to perform to the limit (or as near as possible) of their speed capability in adulthood.

Activities must be fun and not overly technical, particularly for 7–11-year-olds. From a sports perspective, the drills and practices selected must be those that develop foundation skills and physiological development. The former Eastern European countries used to follow such a practice. They ensured that their children were 'physically literate' – able to run effectively, jump and throw. Such a practice is also followed in Australia. These fundamental skills can then be developed in later life and targeted towards certain sports.

Growth spurts

As a coach, teacher or parent working with children you need to be aware of growth spurts. These are times in their lives when they will be less coordinated, for example, due to the way their body and limbs are rapidly growing. Sports coaches are often advised to keep a record of a child's weight and height on a monthly basis, to work out when these growth spurts are occurring – although in most cases it will be obvious. It is important to remember, as a teacher or coach, that a child has not suddenly become a bad player or poor athlete overnight, rather they are trying to coordinate a body that in some cases, and in terms of the performance of certain skills, has a 'mind of its own'. Limbs that were once able to move with relative precision now become gangly, rangy appendages that won't coordinate. It is therefore crucial that you work carefully with children at these times and don't tell them off. You should also try to select drills that will be less taxing – referring to the skill windows will prove a good starting point.

developing speed, endurance and strength

You'll see in table 1 that for boys there is only one aerobic (steady-paced, long-lasting activity) development period that begins at the age of 13. The reasons for this are complex and beyond the scope of this book. Basically, 7–11 year olds should have near boundless stop-start (anaerobic) energy – as anyone who has young children will know. This means that they will naturally increase their anaerobic endurance capacity to a significant extent as they mature. Aerobically they do not possess the right enzymes* to train responsively for this until puberty. The majority of children under 13 therefore find it difficult to sustain steady-paced running (or similar exercise), which is why generations of children have been discouraged from exercising regularly in adulthood – they relate exercise to the cross country runs they were forced to do at school!

*Enzymes are (normally) proteins that are involved in cellular reactions – different enzymes produce different cellular reactions (also known as 'metabolic pathways').

The development of strength is an issue that comes up regularly with children who participate in sports such as rugby, football and athletics. We have seen a number of parents and coaches try to mimic what adult athletes do, by including strength sessions with weights and gym equipment for children, that will supposedly give them that 'competitive edge'. However, there is a simple golden rule to follow when it comes to developing strength for under 16-year-olds: all strength development should be carried out against bodyweight and through running, throwing and jumping movements with very little, if any, external weight (weight training equipment or free weights).

Table 1	Critical physiological and neuromuscular development times for boys			
Age	Skill	Speed	Strength	Endurance (aerobic)
6	Skill			
7	Skill			
8	Skill			
9		Speed 1		
10		Speed 1		
11		Speed 1		
12		Speed 1		
13			Strength	Aerobic
14		Speed 2	Strength	Aerobic
15		Speed 2	Strength	Aerobic
16		Speed 2	Strength	Aerobic
17			Strength	Aerobic
18			Strength	
19				
20				
21				

Table 2	Critical physiologcal and neuromuscular development times for girls			
Age	Skill	Speed	Strength	Endurance (aerobic)
6	Skill			
7	Skill	Speed 1		
8	Skill	Speed 1		
9	Skill			
10				
11				
12		Speed 2		Aerobic
13		Speed 2	Strength	Aerobic
14		Speed 2	Strength	
15			Strength	
16				
17				
18				
19				
20				
21				

Note: The information provided is for guideline purposes only. No two children will mature at exactly the same rate. The windows identified should not be seen as the only times to develop a child's respective qualities, rather they should be regarded as the most fertile times to do so. Progress, though not so great, can be made at other times.

the 'skill hungry' years

Between the ages of 8–12 a child is most receptive to learning skills (and knowledge). Teach these correctly and the child will become a physically gifted adult. Teach them incorrectly and it will be, at best, difficult to produce optimum performance later in life. 'Stem skills' should, as the name suggests, provide the basis from which more advanced skills can be learned later. You should not introduce hugely complex skills as the child will not be big enough or strong enough to perform them. For example, the key to jumping higher is an effective take-off, where the 'free' (non-take-off) leg is driven forcibly upwards so the thigh is parallel to the ground position and the take-off leg is fully extended behind the body to propel the young person upwards. This is the stem skill that should be taught. No mention should be made of a Fosbury flop high jump technique, until the child is of appropriate age, strength and size and only then if they are training for the high jump. Get the stem skill right and optimum performance of a more complex sporting movement will be much easier to achieve later.

health and safety and child protection

As a responsible adult you have a duty of care to the children you are teaching or coaching. If you are a teacher, youth worker or qualified sports coach you will be aware of this and will be familiar with child protection procedures. If, for example, a young person discloses information of a personal nature, you may have to act. Schools and sports clubs should have an appropriate person to whom you can take your concerns.

For more information on child protection in the sports environment, advice and guidelines go to the NSPCC website:

www.nspcc.org.uk/inform/cpsu/cpsu_wda57648.html

making training sessions safe but fun

These days, health and safety has an ever-expanding influence on our daily lives. Coaching all sports at all levels is now increasingly subject to health and safety policy – imposed, for example, by the government, local authority and sports governing bodies. Sports centres and school facilities, for example, must be up to standard to host events and training sessions. As a teacher/coach it will be your job to ensure that the environment you are working in is safe and the equipment you are using is fit for purpose. You may go to the same venue day after day, but you must always view your coaching set-up with fresh eyes. Don't assume that what was safe yesterday will be so today. Also be mindful of weather conditions – if it is raining, the playground or outdoor sports area might be slippery so it would be better to avoid drills and activities that require quick turns and jumps, if an indoor area is not available.

Likewise you should ensure that all the children have the right kit for training and that you know about any medication they may need (for example, asthma pumps). It goes without saying that you, the school or the club/facility should have the contact details of all those you are coaching.

planning your session

The drills in this book have been organised in a way that will help you plan your sessions. There are sections for warm-ups, individuals and groups, reaction and acceleration, agility, body awareness and peripheral vision. You should plan your sessions so that there is a natural progression from warm-up, through to gradually more demanding drills. On one level, in each workout, this should move from warm-up to lower intensity drills, then on to medium and higher intensity drills. For more focused intense training, you could have a block of workouts focusing on one element through a series of sessions. You might have four sessions planned to focus on agility, for example. Select the most appropriate drills from the book and introduce them into four separate planned workouts. Perhaps start with a session that covers agility drills for individuals, such as twisting and turning, and zigzags. Move on to two sessions focusing on group agility, and then introduce ball skills into the final session. The progression should allow the children to develop basic movement skills and get familiar with them, before they perform the more complex drills.

It is always a good idea to include some games and these are best introduced at the end of the session. Many of our drills are in fact games or games-based, such as the bean-bag steal (drill 95). The children will have great fun doing these and normally put in lots more effort. Games will be particularly relevant when working with the 7–11 age range where listening to lengthy explanations is more of an issue.

Timings

If you are working with 30 children and you have set up a drill where each runs for 10 seconds and then stops, the last person will be waiting around for the best part of five minutes before they have a go, and they will have just four runs in the whole session! To get the most out of the session and to keep the children focused, you need to plan for them to be working every 30 to 50 seconds. This means introducing more stations and placing them in groups, usually of four or five.

When looking at timings, you should decide on the aims of your session, the time you have available and the number of children in the group. Once you have done this, you should use our sample session structure below as a guide. This will help the children get the most fun and benefit from their workout.

Length of session:	45–60 min
Warm-up:	6–8 min
Medium intensity drills:	10 min
High intensity drills:	10 min
Games:	12–20 min
Warm down:	5 min

If you have time for a longer session then include more games. Select drills from the relevant sections in the book according to your session aims.

Recovery between drills

When running a session you'll want the children to have enough time to recover from one drill before they start on the next, but you don't want to keep them hanging around so that they get bored and start being disruptive.

For the 7–11 age range roughly proportion the drill and recovery elements in a ratio of 1:4 or 1:5. Most drills take a matter of seconds, so recovery periods will not need to be that long. For example, if an exercise takes 10 seconds to complete, then the rest period should be about 40 seconds. However, if you incorporate some of the games into your workout (see section 9, page 95), then the recoveries could end up being too long. So keep the physically demanding games for the latter parts of your session, and make sure you provide sufficient recovery between them, while also keeping the children interested and having fun.

grading drills for inclusion in a session

We have given each drill an intensity ranking – low, medium and high. This signifies the physical (and mental) demands they make on the children. Drills should progress from low to high intensity across a session, and from session to session in terms of progression. Obviously don't select high intensity drills for the warm-up, but work up to these in the main part of the session. Note: the 'progressions' section of some of the drills may be of a different (usually higher) intensity than the original drill.

equipment

The majority of the drills described in this book can be performed in any location, for example, sports halls, playing fields and athletics tracks.

The basic items of equipment you will need are:

Batons
Bibs
Bean-bags
Canes (preferably multi-coloured)
Cones
Chalk
Foam balls
Hoops (preferably multi-coloured)
Jelly balls (these are made of a material that compresses when it hits the floor)
Low foam/soft hurdles
Light medicine balls: 2-4 kg
Mats
Pen and paper
Quoits
Relay batons
Rugby balls
Stop-watch

Size 4 and size 5 footballs
Tape measure
Tennis balls
Whistle

Most schools, sports clubs and sports centres will have the items of equipment listed. However, if you need to, you'll find suppliers in a quick search on the internet.

WARMING UP

Warming up is crucial for a number of reasons:

1) to get the child ready physically,
2) to get the child ready mentally, and
3) to develop skills that will be used in the main part of the session.

Adults often believe that stretching is an important aspect of the warm-up. It isn't really, as stretching has little to do with preparing muscles for dynamic physical activity. In any case, children tend to naturally possess a far greater range of movement around their joints. For example, a typical stretch for the hamstrings (the muscles at the back of the legs) by bending down to touch the toes with straight legs, has little real application in running and injury prevention. Children, particularly pre-teens, are less likely to pull (or to be technically correct, 'strain') muscles compared to adults in any case. It appears that it is a muscle's inability to cope with the forces that it is subject to that leads to muscle strain – but this should not be an issue with the 7–11-year-olds in your care.

The warm-up drills in this section prepare the child progressively. They build up in intensity and develop a range of movement and strength across the child's body that will specifically prepare muscles, tendons and ligaments for activity.

The warm-up will also switch on all the physiological functions necessary for exercise. Raising body temperature by playing low intensity games, for example, will increase the viscosity of muscles, increase blood flow around the body and get the heart and lungs ready to supply a greater amount of oxygen to the muscles, to fuel activity.

Mentally, the warm-up is also important as it introduces discipline and gets the children thinking about what they are going to be doing in the main part of the session.

warming down

At the end of your session you should organise a short warm-down section. With the 7–11 age group a short period of jogging or walking will suffice. Doing this in the school environment will also be useful as it will calm the children and prepare them for their classroom lessons.

warm-up drills – the cv component

It is important to warm the heart, lungs and muscles up with some gentle cardiovascular (cv) activity. This will increase the viscosity of muscles, making them more stretchy, and will prepare the heart and lungs for exercise.

All the drills in this section should be performed at a low to medium intensity.

drill 1 running

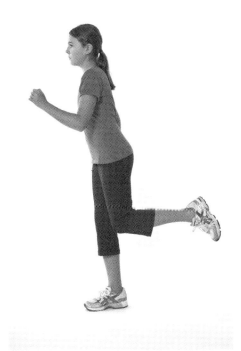

Objective: Running/jogging up and down warm-up

Equipment: Cones

Description: Ask the children to form a line and jog up and down between two cones placed 20m apart.

Coaching points: It's a warm-up, not a race!

Variation: If the children have grasped running sideways and backwards, along with skipping movements, these can be included in the warm-up laps (see sections 3 and 7 in particular). They could jog 20m from the first to the second cone, turn back and perform a drill to the first cone, jog back again to the second cone, keeping going for 2–3 minutes. Keep everything moving by calling out the different movements.

Do: 2–3 minutes.

Intensity: Low

dynamic warm-up drills

The drills that follow are designed to warm up the children's joints in a fun, but functional way.

drill 2 overhead ball pass

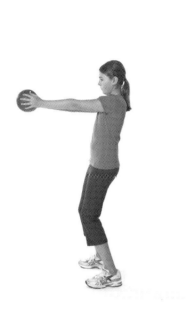 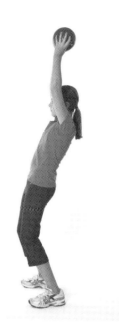

Objective: To warm up the trunk and arms

Equipment: Footballs, or medicine or jelly ball

Description: Ask the children to get into straight lines (ideally you'll need 6–10 in each line). Try to leave at least a metre between each line.

   The child at the back of the line runs to the front carrying the football. They stop and pass it over their head to the person behind and so on down the line. The child at the end runs to the front of the line with the ball and the process starts again. Continue until everyone has run to the front at least once.

Coaching points: Children must stand tall and reach up high as they pass the ball.

Variation: Instead of overhead, change to a sideways turn of the trunk with the ball held in both hands at arms' length to pass the ball behind. The next child rotates in the other direction to pass the ball behind them. Ensure there is sufficient space between the children to avoid contact with each other.

Do: Six times

Intensity: Low

drill 3 — ball pass with trunk rotation around circle

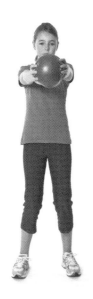 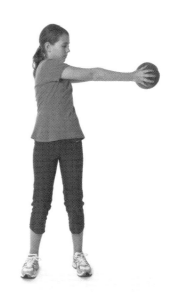

Objective: To warm up the trunk

Equipment: Football or jelly ball

Description: Form a circle. A good way to do this is to get the children to link hands, with their arms outstretched at shoulder height and then ask them to step back as far as they can without breaking the chain. Children should face out and stand with their feet shoulder-width apart. Give the ball to the person at 12 o'clock in the circle. They pass it, using two hands, to the person on their right who takes the ball at arm's length, rotates and passes it on to the person next to them. Continue until the ball is passed around the circle. Change the direction of the pass once the ball is back to where it started.

Coaching points: Encourage rotation of the hips as well as the torso as the ball is passed. Arms should be kept as long as possible.

Variation: Blow a whistle to change the direction of the ball at any point. The speed can also be increased.

Do: Four circles to the left and to the right.

Intensity: Low

drill 4   high knee walk

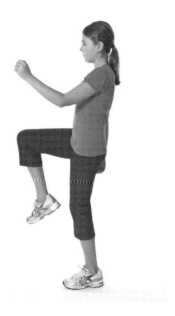 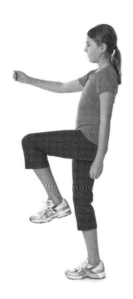

Objective: To develop balance, coordination, strength and a feel for correct running form

Description: Ask the children to walk forwards lifting each leg in turn so that their thigh is parallel to the ground. They should coordinate their arms with their legs – that's opposite arm to leg – bringing their hands in line with their eyes to the front of their body. Elbows should be swung back, behind the body until the upper arm is parallel (or near parallel) to the ground.

Coaching points: Encourage an upright posture. There may be a tendency to lean back when lifting the knees to the required height. You may find that the children have difficulty coordinating opposite arm and leg. A fun way to get this across is to show them what they would look like if they walked swinging the same arm forwards (rather than back) in time with the same leg!

Do: Four sets of 10–15m.

Intensity: Low

drill 5 lunge walk

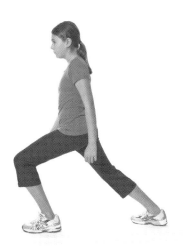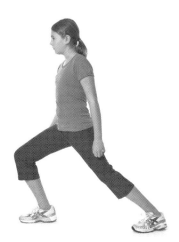

Objective: To develop hip mobility, leg strength and arm-leg coordination

Description: The children stand in a line and each take a big step forwards, placing one foot flat on the floor. Their weight is supported on the toes of their other leg and its knee should be close to the ground. From this lunge position they step into another lunge as they progress forwards.

Coaching points: Encourage an elevated chest and coordination of opposite arm to leg.

Do: Four sets of 10 lunges.

Intensity: Low

drill 6 arm circles

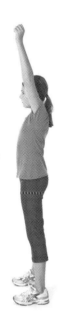 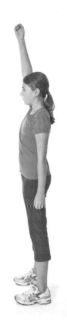

Objective: Dynamic warm-up for the shoulders

Description: The children stand tall with one arm stretched straight up by their heads. They circle this arm back, round, past their head and back to the starting position, reaching up as high as they can with their arm.

Coaching points: Build up speed slowly. The children should maintain a slight bend at the elbow and they should look forwards throughout. Key coaching phrase: 'Brush your ears with your arms'.

Do: Four sets of 10 repetitions.

Variations:
1. Take both arms around at the same time
2. Change the direction of the swings
3. Take one arm backwards and the other forwards (always causes laughter!)

Intensity: Low

drill 7 leg swings

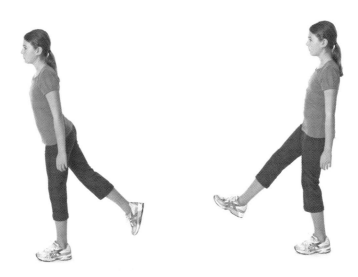

Objective: Dynamic warm-up for the legs

Description: Ask the children to line up and then walk forwards, swinging one leg at a time (with control) to a position in front of their body.

Coaching points: It is important that the drill is performed with control. The torso should remain fairly rigid when the legs are being swung backwards and forwards.

Do: Four sets of 15 m (or four sets of 10 standing leg swings on each leg – see variation).

Variation: The drill can be performed from standing, using a wall or rail for balance. This allows greater emphasis to be placed on swinging the leg back behind the hips.

Intensity: Low

drill 8 leg cycling

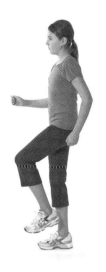 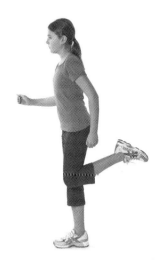

Objective: To develop the running leg action, balance and coordination

Equipment: Wall or rail

Description: The children should stand tall, side-on to a wall or rail, placing their inside hand on it for balance. They should lift the outside thigh to a position parallel to the ground and ideally lift up on the tiptoes of their standing leg. Then they should extend the foot away from the body and sweep it down, round and under, before pulling through to the start position (this completes one leg cycle). Complete a set number of cycles and repeat with the other leg.

Coaching points: As with the leg swing drill, the children should resist the temptation to lean back. It is also important to stress the need for a strong torso and not to yield to the movement of the legs.

Do: Four sets of 10 repetitions on each leg.

Intensity: Low

drill 9 'T'-stretch

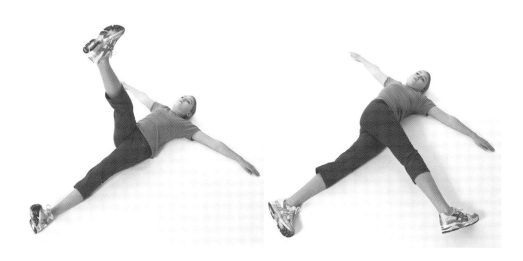

Objective: Lower back, hamstrings and hip stretch (will also develop core strength)

Description: Ask the children to lie on their backs, with their arms outstretched and the backs of their hands on the floor in line with their shoulders to form a 'T' shape. They should lift one leg straight up towards their head. At the sticking point (the limit to their range of movement), they rotate the leg across their body in an attempt to touch the outstretched hand on the opposite side. When their shoulder lifts from the floor, they should pause and then bring the leg back to the centre, before slowly lowering it to the ground. Their other leg should remain pressed into the ground.

Coaching points: Some children will be able to touch their hands with their feet, others will have more difficulty. Keep an eye on all abilities. Regardless of range of movement, the drill should be performed rhythmically and with control.

Do: Three sets of 10 repetitions to each side.

Intensity: Low

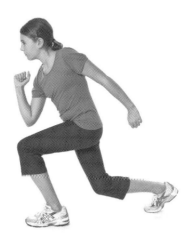

Objective: To warm up and strengthen the hips, hamstrings and bottom muscles

Description: Ask the children to line up. Each should take a big step forwards into a lunge. They then extend their trunk forwards over their thigh and push the elbow (on the same side as the extended foot) down towards the knee or ankle. Then they pause for a second, pull their trunk back to upright and then lunge forwards and repeat the exercise on the other side.

Coaching points: The drill should be performed with control, and balance becomes a big factor.

Do: Four repetitions over 10–20m.

Intensity: Low

drill 11 jog with forward arm circling

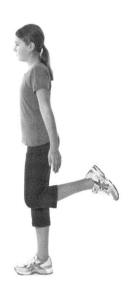 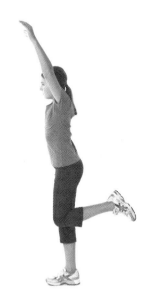

Objective: To develop agility, coordination and shoulder mobility

Description: Ask the children to line up and jog forwards while circling their arms forwards around their heads.

Coaching points: Start slowly then speed up. Encourage an upright posture while making big circles with the arms.

Do: Two sets of 20m.

Intensity: Low

drill 12 kneeling press-ups

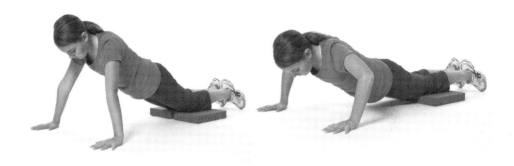

Objective: To develop conditioning and strength for children using their bodyweight.

Description: Working in pairs one child kneels on a mat with their hands on the floor, shoulder-width apart and elbows bent. They should pivot on their knees. To complete the exercise they push up until their arms are straight and then lower back to the starting position with control.

Coaching points: The children should keep the head aligned with the torso.

Do: Five sets of 10 press-ups alternating with their partner.

Intensity: Medium

drill 13 full press-ups

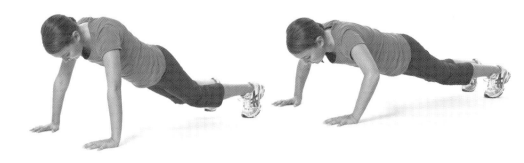

Objective: To develop conditioning and upper body strength

Description: Working in pairs, the children get into a prone position. Placing their hands beneath their shoulders, they push back with their arms to lift their body from the floor. Their legs should be straight behind them, with their weight supported through their toes.

Coaching points: The children should lower their chest to the floor keeping the body straight.

Do: Five sets of 10 press-ups alternating with their partner.

Intensity: Medium/high

AGILITY

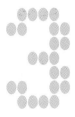

Agility can be defined as the ability to move quickly and fluidly in various directions. It is characterised by light, fast feet and body movements. The drills in this section will develop this skill. Improved agility will benefit all sports and martial arts, as well as dance.

drill 14 backward running

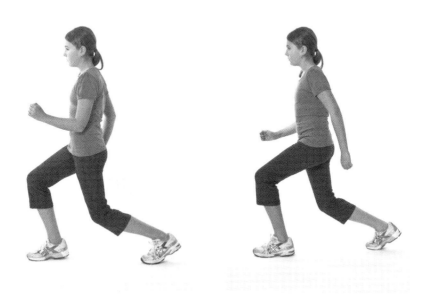

Objective: To develop agility, coordination and leg strength.

Description: The child stands facing backwards to the direction of effort. They run backwards by pushing off from the balls of the feet while taking short steps.

Coaching points: Emphasise that the children should be 'light on their feet'. Arms should be coordinated with legs – opposite arm to leg. When teaching this drill for the first time, stress the need to go slowly. If you are working with a group, set the children off one at a time, or put them into groups of four and make sure they are well spread out to avoid potential collisions. Make sure there are no hazards behind the children which may cause them to trip.

Do: Four sets of 15m.

Intensity: Low

drill 15 sideways skips

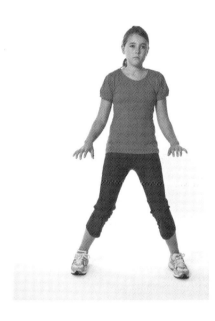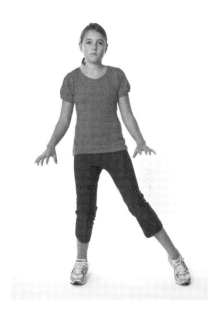

Objective: To develop lateral agility

Description: The child stands sideways on, their feet shoulder-width apart. They bend their knees slightly. The movement is made by pushing from the balls of the feet to skip using a low trajectory sideways. Arms hould be relaxed.

Coaching points: As with backwards running (drill 4), it is important that the young person is light on their feet. Emphasise the importance of quick, light, dynamic steps – 'left, right, left'.

Do: Four sets of 10m (two to the left and two to the right).

Intensity: Low

drill 16 'X' steps (carioca)

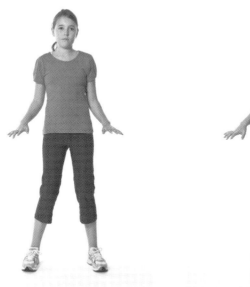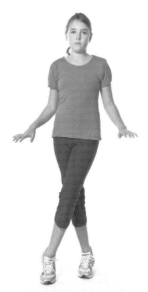

Objective: To develop agility, coordination and quick legs

Description: The child stands sideways on, their feet just beyond shoulder-width apart. One leg is taken in front of the line of the body (passing the outside foot) and then immediately pulled behind what was the outside foot, using very short steps – this creates a crossing movement. It is repeated to move sideways. The child should rotate the core and arms in time with the legs, with the arms held roughly parallel to the ground.

Coaching points: This drill will prove a challenge to the children! Go through the drill slowly, step by step, so that they pick up the required movement. In coaching terminology this is called 'chunking'. In time the children will be able to put all the chunks together.

Do: Four sets of 20m.

Variation: Increase the speed of the drill.

Intensity: Low

drill 17 triangle hops

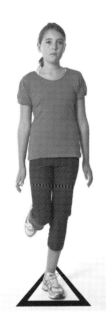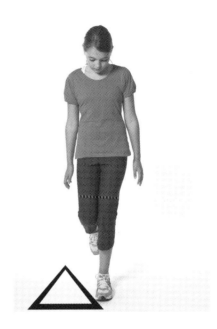

Objective: To develop single leg agility and coordination

Equipment: Tape (depending on location)

Description: Using the lines on a sports hall floor or running track or with tape, mark a triangle. The child hops forwards into the triangle, then out again to the other side and back to the start position. The hops should be performed with a low trajectory.

Coaching points: Encourage the children to be quick and light on their feet. They should use the balls of their feet. The hopping path is that of a right angle triangle.

Do: Four sets of 10 (two sets on each leg).

Variation: Increase the speed.

Intensity: Medium

drill 18 scissor shuffle

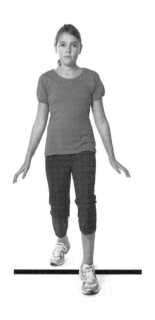 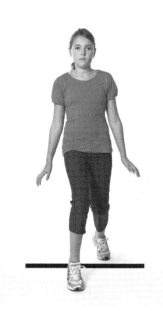

Objective: To develop agility and coordination

Description: Using the lines on a sports hall floor or running track, and working in pairs, one child works while the other rests. Standing with one foot in front and one foot behind a line the child shuffles backwards and forwards across the line for 20 seconds (this is achieved by quick changes of legs – left foot forward, left foot back, right foot forward, right foot back).

Coaching points: Children should use the balls of the feet and take small steps just crossing the line, not too high or too quickly.

Do: Five sets of 20 seconds.

Progression: Work faster

Intensity: Medium

drill 19 bench jogging

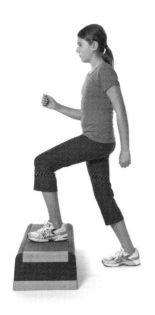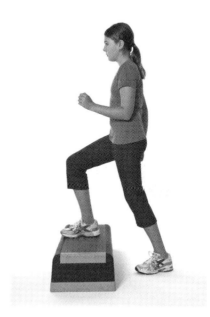

Objective: To develop fitness and agility

Equipment: Bench

Description: The children start by standing in front of a low, sturdy bench or step. When you tell them, they step on and off the bench, alternating between their left and right feet (up on the right, step down with the right, up on the left, step down with the left).

Coaching points: The children should be light on their feet and should keep their chest elevated, coordinating their arms and legs.

Do: Five sets of 30 seconds.

Intensity: Low

drill 20 bench straddle jumps

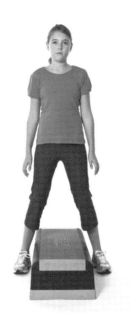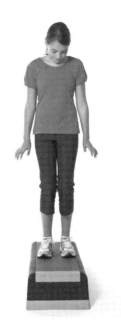

Objective: To develop fitness and agility

Equipment: Step/bench

Description: The children start with their legs astride the bench or step. When you tell them, they jump up and down off the bench quickly – this is achieved by bringing both feet together onto the bench.

Coaching points: Emphasise light contact with the bench and springy movements.

Do: Five sets of 10 jumps.

Intensity: Medium

drill 21 single leg balance with eyes closed

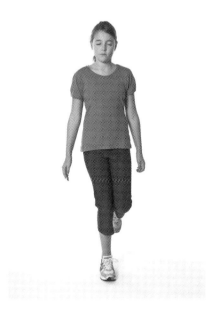

Objective: To develop balance

Equipment: Blindfold (optional)

Description: The children work in pairs. They start by standing on their right leg with eyes closed (or wearing a blindfold) trying to keep their balance for 30 seconds.

Coaching points: Spread the children out so that there is no chance of them knocking each other over if they stumble. Try to get them to relax when performing the drill and to balance naturally.

Do: Five sets of 30 seconds on each leg.

Variation: Run this drill as a competition and see who can hold their balance for the longest time. The child not performing the drill should gently prod the balancing child to further challenge their balance.

Intensity: Low

drill 22 crossover shuffle

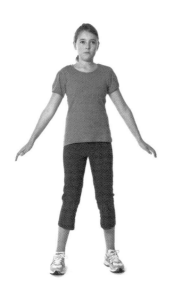 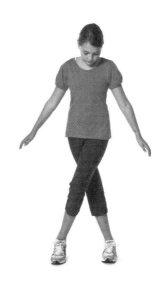

Objective: To develop agility and coordination

Description: Working in pairs, one child works while the other rests. The child crosses their legs, left over right and right over left in a rhythmical movement for 20 seconds on the spot. Their partner then repeats the movement.

Coaching points: The children should work on the balls of their feet, taking small steps just crossing the mid-line of the body. The movement should not be performed too quickly.

Do: Five sets of 20 seconds with the children alternating.

Variation: Work faster.

Intensity: Medium

drill 23 ankle jumps

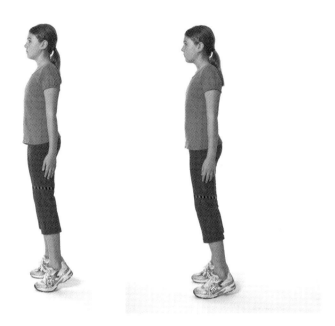

Objective: To develop agility and coordination

Description: The children stand in parallel lines. They should keep their legs straight and jump forwards just using their ankles and feet, i.e. from straight legs.

Coaching points: The hops should be low and rhythmical with the landing kept light.

Do: Five sets of 5m with 60 seconds rest in between.

Intensity: Medium

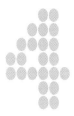

JUMPING

Jumping is a fun activity and, like agility, is a key aspect of most sports. These drills will teach the fundamental principles of good jumping in an enjoyable way.

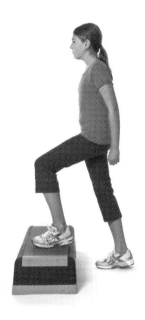 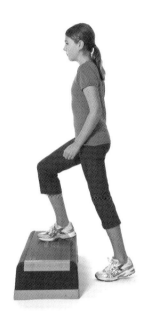

Objective: To develop jumping agility, speed, and strength

Equipment: Box, bench or step 16cm–24cm high

Description: The child starts with one foot on the box and one foot on the floor. On command, they quickly switch the position of their feet on and off the box and continue to do so as quickly as they can for 10 seconds.

Coaching points: The children should move quickly, just touching the top of the box with the balls of their feet. Beware of them hitting the box too hard as this slows them down.

Do: Six sets of 10 seconds with 90 seconds rest in between.

Intensity: Medium

drill 25 double leg box jump

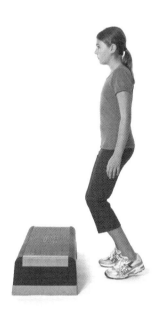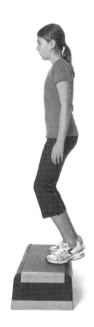

Objective: To develop agility, speed and strength

Equipment: Box, bench or step 16cm–24cm high

Description: The child starts with both feet on the ground in front of the box. On command, they jump up and down, on and off the box as quickly as possible for 10 secs using double leg jumps.

Coaching points: The children should move quickly, just touching the top of the box with the balls of their feet. Beware of them hitting the box too hard as this will slow them down. They should be light on their feet.

Do: Six sets of 10 seconds with 90 seconds rest in between.

Variation: Use a bigger step or box, and do sets of 15–20 seconds.

Intensity: Medium

drill 26 lateral double leg box jump

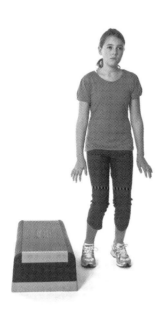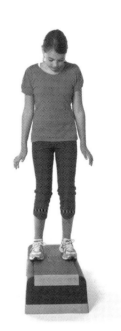

Objective: To develop jumping agility, speed and strength

Equipment: Box, bench or step 16cm–24cm high

Description: The child starts with both feet on the ground, sideways on to the box. On command they jump up and down, on and off the box as quickly as possible for 10 seconds. They then change over to the other side of the box and jump in the same way from that position.

Coaching points: The child should move quickly, just touching the top of the box with the balls of their feet. Beware of them hitting the box too hard as this slows them down. They should be light on their feet.

Do: Ten sets of 10 seconds with 90 seconds rest in between, five sets each side.

Variation: Use a bigger step or box and/or perform for longer, say 15–20 seconds.

Intensity: Medium

drill 27 90 degree double leg box jump

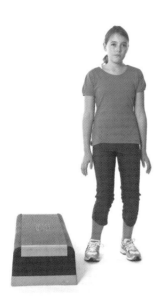 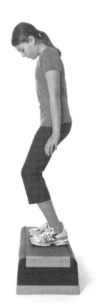

Objective: To develop agility, speed, strength

Equipment: Box, bench or step 16cm–24cm high

Description: The child starts with both feet on the ground, standing sideways on to the box. On command, they jump up and turn through 90 degrees to land on top of the box. They then jump down, turning back through 90 degrees again. The drill is completed quickly for 10 seconds. They then change over to the other side of the box and perform the drill from there.

Coaching points: The child should move quickly, just touching the box with the balls of their feet. Beware of them hitting the box too hard as this will slow them down. Landings should be light and the arms swung to assist the jumps.

Do: Ten sets of 10 seconds with 90 seconds rest in between (five sets each side).

Variation: Use a bigger step or box and/or perform for longer, say 15–20 seconds.

Intensity: Medium

drill 28 single leg box jump

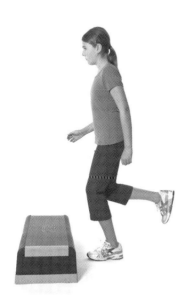 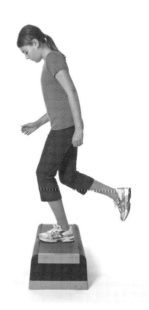

Objective: To develop jumping agility, speed, strength and power

Equipment: Box, bench or step 16cm–24cm high

Description: The child stands on one leg in front of the box. On command, they jump up and down off the box as quickly as possible for 10 seconds on one leg. They rest for 20 seconds and repeat with the other leg.

Coaching points: The child should move quickly, but must place all of their foot on the box. They should keep their chest up and try to maintain a relatively straight body position throughout the drill.

Do: Six sets of 10 seconds with 90 seconds rest between sets.

Variation: Use a bigger step or box and/or perform for longer, say 15–20 seconds.

Intensity: Medium

drill 29 lateral single leg box jump

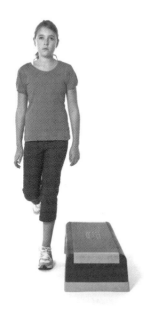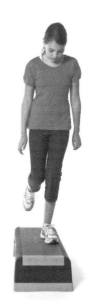

Objective: To develop speed, strength and power

Equipment: Box, bench or step 16cm–24cm high

Description: The child stands on one foot at the side of the box. On command, they quickly jump up and down off the box sideways as quickly as possible for 10 seconds. They rest for 20 seconds, walk to other side of the box or turn through 180 degrees, and repeat with the other leg.

Coaching points: The child should move quickly, but must place all their foot on the box for landings. The chest should be elevated and the body long.

Variation: Use a bigger step or box and/or perform for longer, say 15–20 seconds.

Do: Six sets of 10 seconds with 90 seconds rest in between sets.

Intensity: Medium

sideways alternate double leg box jump

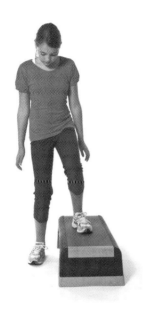 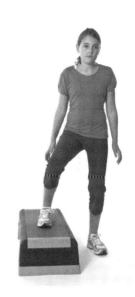

Objective: To develop jumping agility, speed, strength and power

Equipment: Box, bench or step 16cm–24cm high

Description: The child stands with one foot on the box and the other on the ground to the side of the box. On command, they quickly jump over the box, to place the other leg on the ground and the other on the box, they then jump back over the box and repeat for 10 seconds. They rest for 20 seconds and repeat with the right leg.

Coaching points: The children should move quickly, touching the ball of the foot on the box. Beware of them hitting the step too hard as this slows them down.

Do: Six sets of 10 seconds with 90 seconds rest in between sets.

Intensity: Medium

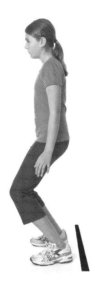 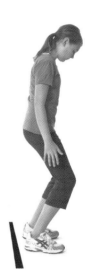

Objective: To develop jumping agility and coordination

Description: Working in pairs, one child works while the other rests. The child stands with both feet behind a line, they jump and turn through 180 degrees to the right, land on both feet and hold for 3 seconds. They then jump up again and turn though 180 degrees to the left to land again on both feet.

Coaching points: The child jumps high enough to be able to turn and to land 'lightly' on the balls and heels of their feet. They should swing their arms to assist the jump and turn.

Do: Ten sets of two jumps then change over.

Intensity: Medium

high agility jump

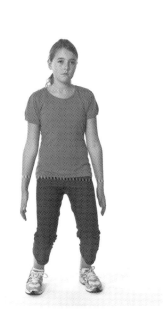
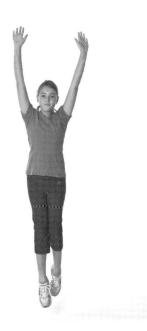

Objective: To develop agility and coordination

Equipment: Wall

Description: Working in pairs. The child stands close to a wall, bends their knees and jumps as high as they can to touch the wall at the highest point of their reach. Rest for 5 seconds and repeat.

Coaching points: The child should swing their arms to assist their jump and land lightly on both feet. They should flex (bend) their knees slightly to control the landing.

Do: Five sets of 5 jumps alternating with their partner after every set.

Intensity: Medium

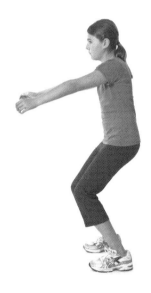
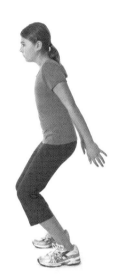

Objective: To develop jumping strength

Equipment: Mat or long jump pit

Description: Work in pairs. The child stands with feet shoulder-width apart in a semi-squat position on the edge of the pit/mat and jumps as far as possible.

Coaching points: The child should jump as high and as long as possible. They should use their arms to add momentum to spring into the jump. The arms should be swung backwards and forwards past the hips and to time with the jump take-off. The child should try to keep their head and chest elevated throughout the jump.

Do: Five sets of 5 jumps alternating with their partner after every set.

Intensity: Medium

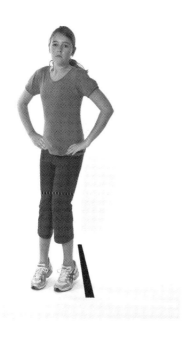 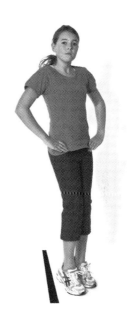

Objective: To develop jumping agility and coordination

Description: Working in pairs. The child jumps and twists their feet and hips left and then right while in the air, landing on the same spot.

Coaching points: The children should work on the balls of their feet and take small steps to just cross the mid-line of the body 'left, right, left', and so on. Jumps should not be too high or performed too quickly.

Do: Five sets of 20 seconds alternating with their partner after every set.

Intensity: Medium

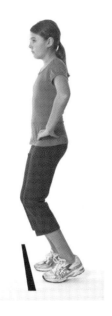 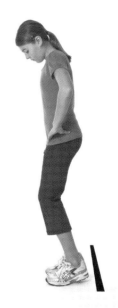

Objective: To develop jumping agility and coordination

Description: Work in pairs. The child stands with both feet behind a line and jumps backwards and forwards across it for 10 seconds.

Coaching points: The children should jump and land on the balls of the feet and use a low trajectory to make the jumps. The arms should be swung backwards and forwards to assist the jump.

Do: Five sets of 10 seconds alternating with partner after every set.

Intensity: Medium

drill 36 double leg lateral jumps

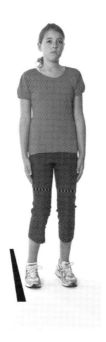 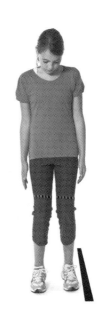

Objective: To develop jumping agility and coordination

Description: Work in pairs. The child stands with both feet facing sideways onto a line. They jump from side to side across it for 10 seconds.

Coaching points: The children should work on the balls of their feet and use a low jump trajectory, keeping toes pointing straight ahead. Their body should remain straight, they should look straight ahead and the landing should be light and reactive.

Do: Five sets of 10 seconds alternating with partner after every set.

Intensity: Medium

drill 37 single leg lateral jumps

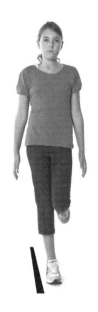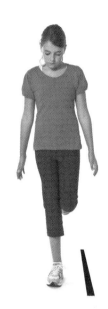

Objective: To develop jumping agility and coordination

Description: Work in pairs. The child stands on one leg facing sideways to a line. They then jump from side to side across the line for 10 seconds. They change legs and repeat.

Coaching points: The children should work on the balls of the feet, using small hops to just cross the line. The jumping foot should face towards the front (parallel to the line) and the torso should be upright.

Do: Five sets of 10 seconds on each leg, alternating with their partner after every set.

Intensity: Medium

single leg jumps forwards and backwards

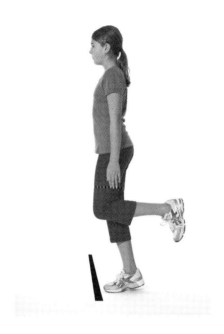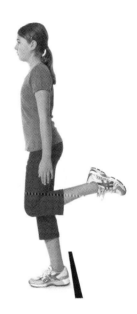

Objective: To develop jump agility and coordination

Description: Work in pairs. The child stands with one foot behind the line. They jump forwards and backwards across the line for 10 seconds.

Coaching points: The child should remain light on their feet and make the landings dynamic. Low trajectory jumps should be made and the arms should be swung backwards and forwards in time with the legs.

Do: Five sets of 10 seconds on each leg before changing over with their partner.

Intensity: Medium

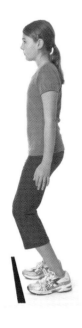 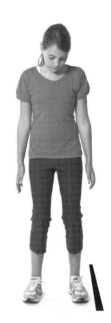

Objective: To develop agility and coordination

Description: Work in pairs. The child stands with both feet behind a line. They then jump up and twist through 90 degrees to the right to land on both feet the other side of the line. They then jump up to twist through 90 degrees to the left (to land where they started), again landing on both feet.

Coaching points: The child should jump high enough to be able to turn through 90 degrees. Landings must be light and dynamic and made on the balls of the feet. The arms should be used to assist the jump and aid rotation.

Do: Ten sets of two jumps, alternating with partner after every set.

Intensity: Medium

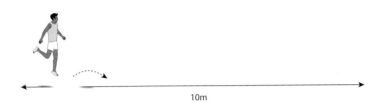

10m

Objective: To develop jumping ability

Description: The children hop over 10m aiming to cover the distance in as few hops as possible.

Coaching points: Encourage a head and chest-up position and a flat-footed landing. The hopping leg should be cycled under the body and brought to the front in preparation for each take-off. Landings should be light and dynamic. Arms should be coordinated with the legs.

Variation: Organise as a race – ensure that the children are sufficiently spaced to avoid collisions.

Do: Four sets of 10m (two sets on each leg).

Intensity: High

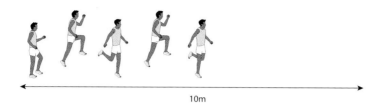

10m

Objective: To develop jumping ability

Description: From a standing position, the child leaps forward to land flat-footed on one leg. They repeat the action immediately and leap onto their other foot. This pattern is continued until they clear the 10m distance.

Coaching points: The child must have an elevated chest with the head looking forwards. They must be encouraged to swing their non-take-off leg forwards powerfully at the take-offs into each step and then hold it for as long as they can before landing on it.

Do: Four sets of 10m.

Intensity: High

standing triple jump
(hop, step and jump)

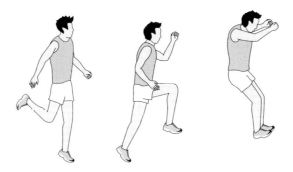

Objective: To develop jumping ability and coordination

Description: From a standing position, the child hops, steps and jumps.

Coaching points: Some children may have difficulty coordinating the triple jump movement. A useful phrase to explain how they should move their legs to perform the three phases is to say, 'same leg, other leg, feet together'. You could also use hoops or draw circles to indicate where each phase should land. The distance between them can be increased as the child learns the triple jump movement. As with all the jumps, an elevated chest and head-up position should be maintained and the arms should balance the flight phase.

Do: Six jumps.

Intensity: High

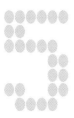

THROWING

Throwing is a vital component of sports such as cricket, athletics, rugby and basketball. When teaching the throwing drills, don't just look at the movement of the arm but that of the whole body. For most of the drills in this section, power will be best produced by engaging the legs and the torso in a sequential manner to release power through the arm or arms. With the single arm throw drills, it's always a good idea to encourage the children to throw with their non-preferred arm as well as their leading arm.

Many of the drills require the thrower's partner to catch the ball, which in itself is a valuable skill.

drill 47 sitting backwards ball throw

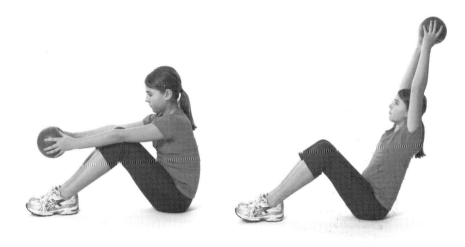

Objective: To develop throwing ability, coordination and teamwork

Equipment: One football per pair

Description: Work in pairs. The child sits on the floor with their knees bent to 90 degrees and their feet flat on the floor. They should hold the sides of the ball. They should face away from their partner who should stand about 4m away. The child throws the ball overhead to their partner, who catches it and then rolls it back (the throwing child will need to turn their head and torso to gather the ball).

Coaching points: The arms need to be kept long and straight during the throw and the child needs to time the velocity and height so their partner can catch it.

Do: Three sets of 10 reps, changing over after each set.

Intensity: Medium

drill 48 single under arm throw

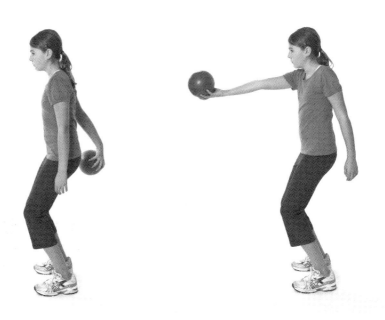

Objective: To develop throwing power and coordination

Equipment: One ball per pair

Description: Work in pairs. The child stands about 1.5m away from a wall with the ball held in their right hand. They should throw the ball underarm against the wall, catch it with the same hand (before it touches the floor) and then throw the ball again. After 10 throws they should repeat with their left arm.

Coaching points: The ball needs to be thrown firmly so that the child can catch it without moving significantly.

Do: Two sets of 10 reps on each side, alternating with the partner after every set.

Intensity: Low

drill 49 Superman throws

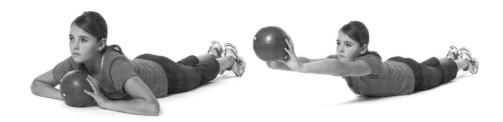

Objective: To develop agility and throwing coordination

Equipment: One ball per pair

Description: Work in pairs. The child lies flat on their stomach holding the ball in two hands and out to the front of their head. Their partner should stand 3m away in front of them. The child raises their torso to throw the ball to their partner who rolls the ball back to them for the next throw.

Coaching points: The drill needs to be performed with control, as the range of movement of the lower back and abdomen will affect the ability of the child to perform the throw.

Variation: Throw the ball with one hand

Do: Four sets of 10 reps each, alternating after each set.

Intensity: Medium

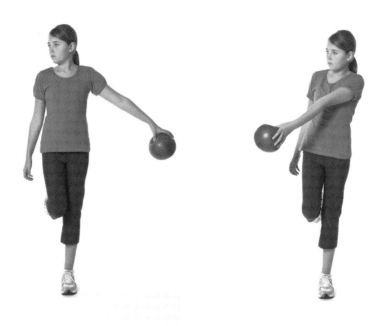

Objective: To develop balance, coordination strength and throwing skill

Equipment: Football or tennis ball and wall

Description: Work in pairs. The child stands on one leg with the foot of the other tucked up towards their bottom. They throw the ball sideways onto the wall, using an underarm throw and catch it while remaining on the one leg – this will test their balance. They do 10 repetitions on one leg and then 10 on the other while throwing the ball with their other hand and facing the wall from the other side. They then swap positions with their partner, who performs the drill.

Coaching points: The child should try and stay balanced on one leg and ensure that they don't throw the ball too hard nor too slowly.

Variation: Use a tennis ball – it will be harder to catch the tennis ball with one hand.

Do: Four sets of 10 reps on each leg, swapping with their partner after each set.

Intensity: Medium

single leg balance and forward throw to partner

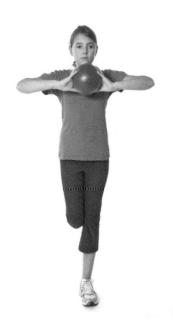 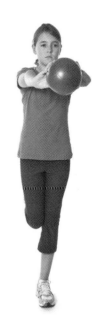

Objective: To develop balance, coordination, strength and throwing skill

Equipment: One football per pair

Description: Work in pairs. The children face each other standing 2m apart. Both should stand on the same leg. They then throw the ball to each other 10 times trying to keep their balance. They should use a chest pass action. They should do 10 repetitions while standing on one leg and 10 on the other.

Coaching points: The children should try and stay balanced on one leg and ensure they don't throw the ball too hard or too slowly.

Do: Four sets of 20 (one set equals 10 reps on each leg).

Intensity: Medium

drill 52   single leg balance and sideways partner throw

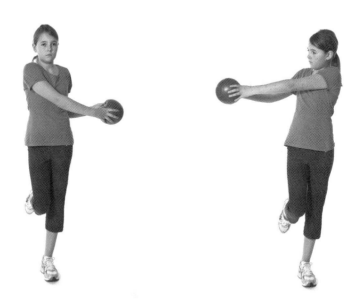

Objective: To develop balance, coordination strength and throwing skill

Equipment: One football per pair

Description: Work in pairs. Both children stand on one leg as described in drill 47. They should be side-on to each other and about 2m apart. They then throw the ball to each other 10 times while trying to keep their balance. They do 10 repetitions on one leg and then 10 repetitions on the other leg.

Coaching points: The children should try and remain balanced and ensure they don't throw the ball too hard or too slowly. The sideways throw will affect the mechanics of their balance and they will have to work that much harder to catch, throw and balance.

Do: Four sets of 20 reps on each leg (one set equals 10 reps on each leg).

Intensity: Medium

drill 53 single leg balance and throw in groups of four

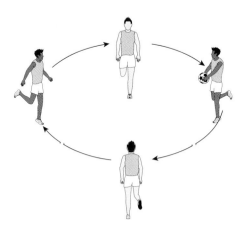

Objective: To develop balance, coordination, teamwork and throwing skill

Equipment: Football

Description: Working in fours, the children stand in a circle – about 2m from each other. They should all stand on the same leg. They then throw the ball to each other, while attempting to maintain their balance. They do 10 repetitions on one leg throwing the ball in a clockwise direction and then 10 in an anti-clockwise direction. They then swap legs and repeat.

Coaching points: The ball should not be thrown too hard nor too slowly to ensure that each child can catch the ball. The ball should be thrown using a chest pass action.

Variation: Play as a competition to see how many times they can throw and catch as a team on one leg, or against the clock.

Do: Four sets of 20 reps (one set equals 10 reps on each leg).

Intensity: Medium

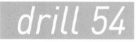
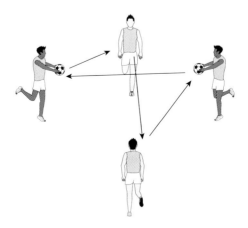

Objective: To develop balance, coordination, teamwork and fitness

Equipment: Two balls

Description: The drill is set up as drill 53, however the children facing each other in the circle throw two balls backwards and forwards between each other 10 times, trying to keep their balance and avoiding hitting the other ball crossing the circle. They do 10 repetitions on one leg and then 10 repetitions on the other leg.

Coaching points: The children should try and stay balanced on one leg while throwing and catching. They should be encouraged to find ways to work together so the balls don't clash.

Do: Four sets of 20 reps (one set equals 10 reps on each leg).

Intensity: Medium

seated forward throws

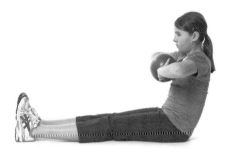 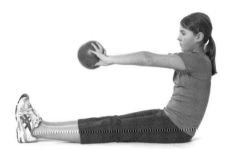

Objective: To develop throwing strength and coordination

Equipment: One football per pair

Description: Work in pairs. The children sit on the floor with their legs straight out in front of them, holding a ball, ready to perform a chest pass. Their partner should stand about 5m in front of them ready to receive the ball. They catch it and roll it back.

Coaching points: The throw comes through the arms and torso.

Do: Four sets of 10 throws, alternating with the partner after each set of 10 throws.

Intensity: Medium

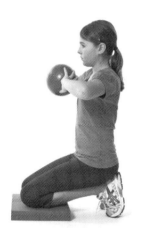 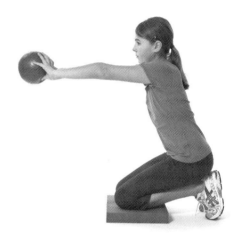

Objective: To develop throwing ability and coordination

Equipment: Football, mats

Description: Work in pairs. Each child kneels on a mat, with one holding a ball, with hands evenly placed to the sides of the ball. Their partner stands 10m away ready to catch the ball. The first child throws the ball to their partner, who rolls it back.

Coaching points: The child should remain on their knees throughout the drill and not topple forwards. They should use their torso to add power to the throw by taking it backwards. They should fully extend their arms when they throw the ball.

Do: Five sets of 10 throws, alternating with the partner.

Intensity: Medium

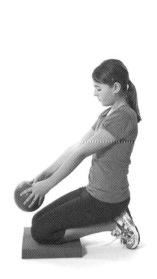
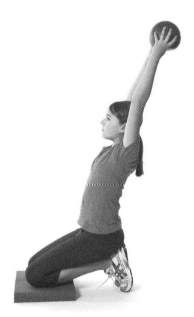

Objective: To develop throwing ability and coordination

Equipment: Football, mat

Description: Work in pairs. The child kneels on a mat, holding the ball. Their partner should stand about 10m behind them, ready to receive the ball. The child throws the ball overhead to their partner who rolls it back.

Coaching points: The child should remain on their knees throughout the drill, and should keep their arms and torso long when they throw the ball. Encourage them to try not to throw the ball too hard initially. They can then learn the best trajectory with which to throw the ball.

Do: Four sets of 10 throws, alternating with the partner.

Intensity: Medium

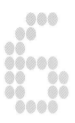

REACTION

Reaction is a great physical ability that is applicable to numerous sports and everyday life. The drills in this section will develop quick, coordinated and strong movements and lay down the foundations for the specific reactive movements required for sport. Reaction drills are also by their nature great fun to do.

follow the leader

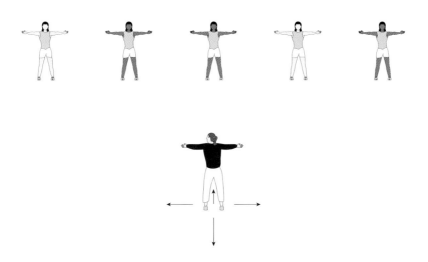

Objective: To develop reaction, agility, fitness and team work

Equipment: About 30–40m of space

Description: Ask the children to form straight lines. They should be facing you and about 5 metres away. If you have more than 10 children in your group, then form two lines, one behind the other, 1m apart. The children have to react to, and mirror, your movements – if you move backwards, the children move forwards; if you go left, they have to move to the right and so on.

Coaching points: The children should aim to move as a team. They should keep their heads up, so they can see what you are doing and they should be light on their feet – making the movements from the balls of their feet. The drill should last for 20–30 seconds.

Do: Four sets with 60–90 seconds rest in between.

Intensity: Medium

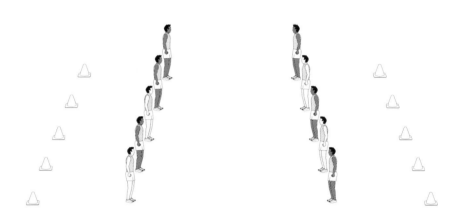

Objective: To develop agility, reaction, fitness and team work

Equipment: 30–40m of space and cones to mark the area

Description: Ask the children to form two straight lines 5m apart and facing each other – Team A and Team B. Mark out a 5m perimeter with cones behind each team. You should use four key words – these are the seasons, 'spring, summer, autumn and winter' – to provide the 'direction' for the teams. On hearing the relevant season the teams react as follows:

Spring: Run backwards 5m (to the cone perimeter) and quickly forwards to the starting position
Summer: Sit down on the floor
Autumn: Turn and run to the cone perimeter and then run back to the starting position, finishing with hands held above heads (reaching for the sky)
Winter: Do five jumps on the spot on two legs and finish standing on one leg

Coaching points: The children should try to move as a team. They need to keep their heads up and listen to your commands. Their movements need to be quick and correct. You should make the session fun by giving everyone time to get back to their line before shouting out another season.

When the drill is performed for the first time the children will need a little more time to get used to the commands. For extra fun you can add some spurious commands such as 'sand', 'sprite', 'work', to see how the children react. You could also make up your own physical reactions for these commands to provide an extra challenge.

Do: Three sets of 3 minutes with 90 seconds rest in between to recover.

Intensity: High

drill 60 ball drop reaction drill

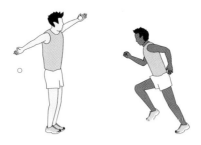

Objective: To develop reaction, fitness and team work

Equipment: About 5m of space, two tennis balls

Description: The children work in pairs. They should face each other standing 3m apart. 'A' holds two tennis balls in the hands of outstretched arms and drops one of the two balls. 'B' reacts and runs to catch the ball before the second bounce.

Coaching points: If the catcher struggles to get to the ball, shorten the distance between the children. Each child should do 10 ball drops, before swapping over.

Do: Four sets of 10 ball drops, alternating roles after each set.

Intensity: High

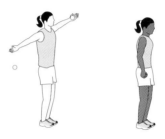

Objective: To develop reaction, fitness and team work

Equipment: About 5m of space, two tennis balls

Description: The children work in pairs. They should stand 2m apart. 'B' should stand with their back to 'A'. 'A' holds two tennis balls in their outstretched arms, and calls out 'left' or 'right' – depending on the ball they decide to drop. On hearing the command, 'B' should turn through 180 degrees, run and try to catch the ball before the second bounce.

Coaching points: If the children are struggling to get to the ball before the second bounce, shorten the distance between them. Do 10 drops each, before swapping positions.

Do: Four sets of 10 ball drops, swapping positions and roles after each set.

Intensity: High

drill 62 ball reaction and sprint

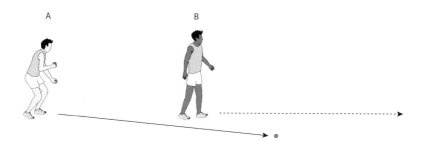

A   B

Objective: To develop reaction, fitness and team work

Equipment: About 5m of space, two tennis balls

Description: Work in pairs. 'A' is the 'server'. They should hold a tennis ball in the hands of each of their outstretched arms. 'B' faces away from 'A' about 3m away. 'A' then rolls one of the tennis balls to the right or left of 'B', who reacts and chases the ball, catches it, picks it up and then runs back to the starting position before returning the ball to 'A'.

Coaching points: 'B' should time the pace of the ball so that it's not too fast and not too slow in terms of allowing 'A' to reach it. Do 10 repetitions before swapping positions.

Do: Four sets of 10 ball drops, swapping positions and roles after each set.

Intensity: High

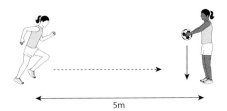

5m

Objective: To develop reaction and explosive first steps

Equipment: Football and cones

Description: Work in pairs. Mark out a distance of 5m with cones. 'A' stands by the first cone and 'B' by the second. 'A' holds the football at shoulder height in two hands and to one side of their body. They then drop the ball. 'B' accelerates and attempts to catch the ball before it bounces for the second time. On catching the ball they then turn and sprint back to the starting position where they roll the ball back to A. Trial and error will be needed to establish the right distance to make the drill most effective within the 5m space.

Coaching points: Stress a snappy first step, with a dynamic leg drive. To establish the optimum distance between the children, the drill can be performed a number of times starting with a smaller gap, with the reacting child gradually moving further away to the point where they can't quite catch the ball.

Do: Four to eight repetitions each.

Intensity: High

kneeling to sprint 10–20m

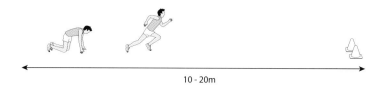

10 - 20m

Objective: To develop reaction and acceleration

Equipment: Cones

Description: The child kneels on all fours. On command, they react, get up and sprint 10–20m from the kneeling position to the cone.

Coaching points: Encourage the first step from the kneeling position to be made with the stronger leg.

Variation: Line the children up so that they can race against each other.

Do: Six repetitions

Intensity: High

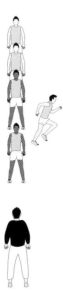

Objective: A fun way to develop reaction and acceleration

Equipment: Tape/cones

Description: Mark out three lines, each 10–15m apart. Line the children up along the centre line. They should face you with their legs astride the line. Your command will either be 'left' or 'right'. On hearing this they will turn and sprint in that direction.

Coaching points: Although there is a high fun element to this drill, stress the importance of quick pushing strides to accelerate rapidly. Spread the children out along the centre line to avoid collisions.

Variations: Change the commands of 'left' or 'right' to a clap and whistle (having told the children which sound indicates left and right).

Do: Ten repetitions.

Intensity: High

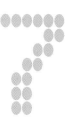

ACCELERATION

Like agility and reaction, acceleration makes for fun drills while developing fitness. Nevertheless, you should try to encourage a good 'driving' body position among the children. They should push back with their legs, with the work being done behind their body. The first drills in this section will develop an awareness of this position.

drill 66 low knee wall runs

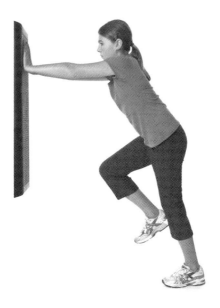

Objective: To develop fitness and acceleration

Equipment: Wall

Description: The children line up facing the wall. They should lean their body forwards and place their hands at shoulder height against the wall (their body should be angled and braced). To your command they should 'run' as if trying to move the wall – lifting their knees 10–16 cm from the ground.

Coaching points: The children should 'run' for 10 seconds without slowing down. They should make ground contact with the balls of their feet.

Do: Five x 10 second runs with 60–90 seconds rest.

Intensity: Medium

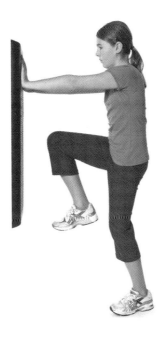

Objective: To develop fitness and acceleration

Equipment: Wall

Description: Assume the same starting position as for the previous drill. This time on your command the children lift their knees so that their thigh is parallel to the ground and run as if to move the wall.

Coaching points: The children should ensure they run for 10 seconds without slowing down – ground contact should be made with the balls of the feet.

Do: Five x 10 second runs, with 60–90 seconds rest.

Intensity: High

drill 68 running in pairs

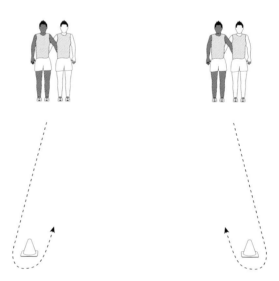

Objective: To develop acceleration, fitness and team work

Equipment: Cones and lots of space

Description: Work in pairs. The children should put their arms around each other's waists. The pairs line up side by side, each facing a cone which is placed 15m in front of them. Space the cones out so that there is sufficient space for each pair to run around their cone. The drill starts on your command, and the pairs must run 20m around their cone to return to the starting position i.e. they must run together in a straight line, to and from their cone.

Coaching points: The children should run as a team, turning together and staying linked around the waist, avoiding collisions with the other pairs.

Do: Four runs with 60–90 seconds rest.

Variation:
1. Do a relay of three teams
2. Hold hands instead of placing arms around waist
3. Increase the number of children in the team.

Intensity: High

standing backward throw with a sprint

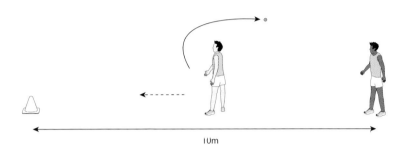

1Um

Objective: To develop acceleration, agility and coordination

Equipment: Football or tennis ball, cones

Description: Work in pairs. 'A' throws the ball upwards and backwards as far as they can. On releasing the ball, they sprint forwards 5m running past a cone. 'B' stands behind 'A' approximately 10m away ready to catch the ball. The idea is to sprint past the cone before their partner catches the ball.

Coaching points: The children must pump their arms and legs as fast as they can when they run to the cone. If you start the pairs off one at a time you can judge whether the child gets past the cone or not, before the ball is caught or hits the ground.

Do: Four sets of 5 throws, alternating positions after every set.

Intensity: High

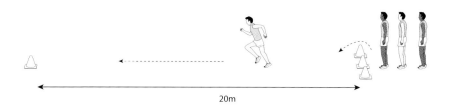

20m

Objective: To develop acceleration

Equipment: Cones and a lot of space

Description: Mark out a distance of 20m with cones and then place three cones evenly spaced apart at the start. Put the children into teams of four or five and get them to stand behind their line of three cones. You can set up as many lines as you have teams (and cones). The first person in the team starts on your command and jumps over the cones, using double leg jumps. They then sprint to the cone placed at 20m and walk back (if there are teams they should turn to the right and walk back). Once they are walking back the next person in the team starts.

Coaching points: The children should make their jumps light and dynamic. On landing from the cone jump, they should pump their arms and legs to accelerate away quickly. Space the teams out.

Do: Four to six runs.

Variation: Turn the drill into a relay race by having members of the team sprint to and round the 20m cone and back to the start, where they hand over to the next runner by touching hands.

Intensity: High

BALANCE AND COORDINATION

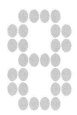

Balance and coordination are skills that are easily transferred both to everyday life and sports performance. Being aware of one's body in space is a vital attribute – this is known as 'kinaesthetic awareness'. It is best that balance drills be performed at the end of a session or early on after the warm-up, otherwise the chances are that the children will be too excitable to perform them at their best.

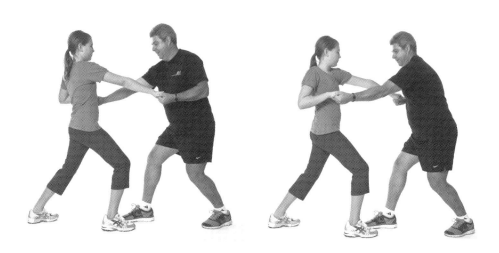

Objective: To develop balance and coordination

Description: The children stand facing each other, holding hands and with their right knees forward. On your command, they should pump their arms backwards and forwards.

Coaching points: The children should not be working so hard that they try to pull each other over. Head should be elevated.

Do: Six sets of 10 seconds with 30 seconds rest between sets.

Intensity: Medium

pumping arms and legs

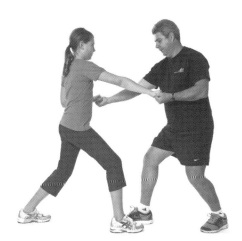 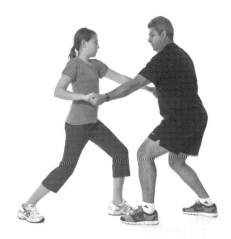

Objective: Coordination, balance and fitness

Description: The children assume the same starting position as for the previous drill. To your command they move their legs and arms alternately – quick-stepping forwards with one leg and back with the other, while pumping their arms backwards and forwards in rhythm for 10 seconds.

Coaching points: The children should remain at arms' length so they have room to move their legs, without hitting each other. As with the previous drill they should not be working so hard that they are trying to pull each other over.

Do: Six sets of 10 seconds with 30 seconds rest in between sets.

Intensity: High

drill 73 leg swings

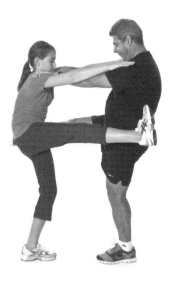 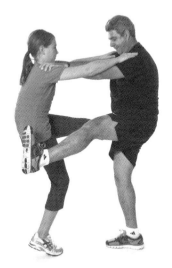

Objective: To develop balance, coordination and agility

Description: The children stand facing each other. They should place their arms on each other's shoulders and stand with their legs shoulder width apart. On your command they should swing their right legs straight up under the left arm of their partner. When their legs return to the ground they should immediately swing their left leg up – this should be done using a quick skipping movement.

Coaching points: The children should remain at arms' length so they have room to move their legs and work together in a rhythm that is neither too fast nor too slow.

Do: Four sets of 10 seconds with 30 seconds rest between sets.

Intensity: High

drill 74 single leg balance

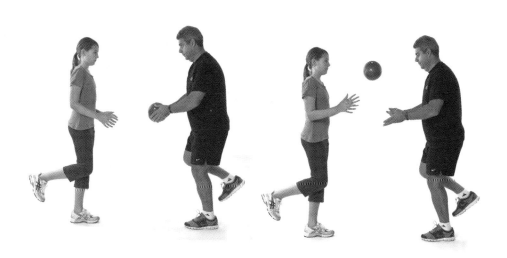

Objective: To develop balance

Equipment: Football or tennis ball

Description: Work in pairs. The children should both stand on one leg facing each other about 2m apart. 'A' holds a football or tennis ball and throws the ball at various angles to 'B' – who tries to keep their balance while they catch and throw the ball back. The children work together to keep their balance and the ball.

Coaching points: 'A' serves at various angles and heights to test 'B', but in a way that they should be able to make the catch.

Do: Six sets of 20 seconds on each leg with the children alternating roles every 40 seconds.

Intensity: Medium

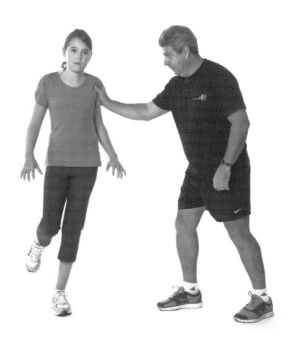

Objective: To develop balance

Description: Pair up the children and have them stand facing each other. 'A' stands on their left leg. 'B' then pushes 'A' against their shoulders – forwards, sideways and from behind – while 'A' tries to keep their balance. The drill continues for 15 seconds, then the children swap positions.

Coaching points: 'A' should slightly bend the knee of their standing leg and engage the core (tense their stomach and back muscles) to help keep their balance and remain rigid. 'B' should not shove 'A' but apply moderate force.

Do: Four sets of 15 seconds on each leg, alternating positions after each child has balanced on their right and left legs.

Intensity: Medium

hop and hold

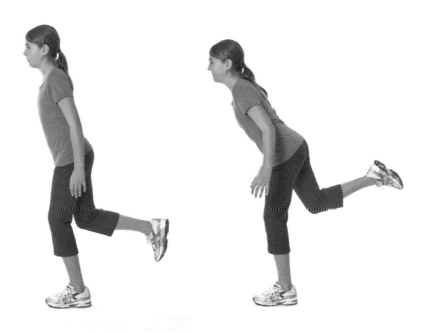

Objective: To develop balance

Description: Get the children into teams of four or more and have them make a small circle. To perform the drill they should all stand on one leg and hop to land on the same leg. The landing is held for 5 seconds. They then walk back to the starting position and change legs to repeat the drill.

Coaching points: The children should try to land and hold their balance; this is best achieved by using a slightly bent knee.

Do: Two sets of 10 repetitions alternating between left and right legs.

Intensity: Medium

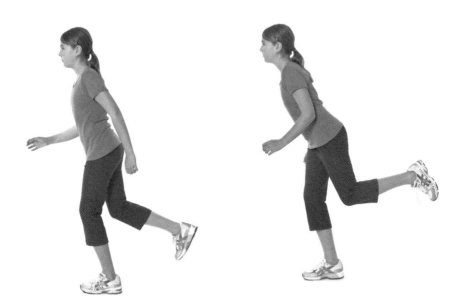

Objective: To develop balance

Description: The young people stand facing each other in a circle in groups of four or more. Standing on the left leg they step and land on their right leg and hold for a count of 5 seconds (you can count out the time). They then walk back to the starting position and change legs.

Coaching points: The children should try to jump at least 0.75–1m on the same leg, while holding their balance on landing. They should land with a slightly bent knee and try to keep their torso up throughout the drill.

Do: Four sets of 10 repetitions alternating starting legs.

Intensity: High

GAMES

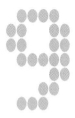

This part of the book is dedicated entirely to enjoyment by focusing on games. The activities involve all the specific components targeted by the drills in the previous sections. It is best to include these at the conclusion of your session.

drill 78 triangle running 1

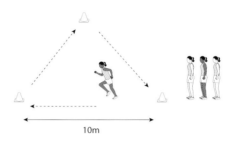

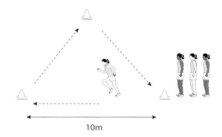

Objective: To develop speed, fitness and agility

Equipment: Cones

Description: Mark two equilateral triangles using the cones. These should be side by side and 2m apart. The triangle's sides should each measure 10m. Each child (or team of children) has a triangle and starts at the same time, running around the triangle in the same direction, as quickly as they can to finish where they started. After a rest they change sides to start on the other side of the triangle to enable them to run in both directions. With teams each runner should start their leg once the person in front of them passes the start cone.

Coaching points: The children should take the corners tightly, using small steps. The work to rest ratio is 1:4. If working with large groups the ideal number is five runners per triangle.

Do: Ten runs each – 5 in each direction (30–60 seconds recovery between runs).

Intensity: High

triangle running 2

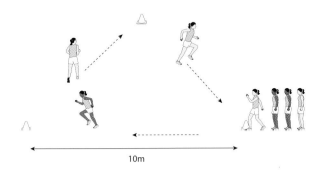

10m

Objective: To develop speed and fitness, and change of direction as a team

Equipment: Cones

Description: Mark out two triangles as with the previous drill. Each should have a team of seven. On your command the first runner in each team starts running around the triangle. The next person starts when the first passes the first cone in their triangle. The teams continue to run around the triangle in this fashion until they have all completed five runs each. After a break, the two teams move to the other side in their respective triangles, so that they run around in the opposite direction.

Coaching points: The children should be alert to what is going on and start at the right time. They should not overtake each other.

Do: Five sets of five runs in each direction (30–60 seconds recovery between runs).

Intensity: High

drill 80 triangle running 3

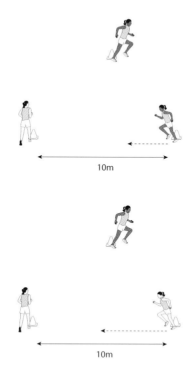

10m

10m

Objective: To develop speed, fitness and change of direction

Equipment: Cones.

Description: Groups of three working, others resting. Mark out a triangle as you have for the previous two drills. Get the children into teams of three, one person on each cone. Each starts running on your command. The children run around the triangle as quickly as they can chasing their team mates and finishing at the position they started at. Then the next three children begin.

Coaching points: The children should try to catch the person in front of them. The direction of the run should be changed after each repetition. To control the running intervals you can use your arm as a barrier to start the young people off at the designated time.

Do: Eight runs, four in each direction.

Intensity: High

triangle running 4 'in and out'

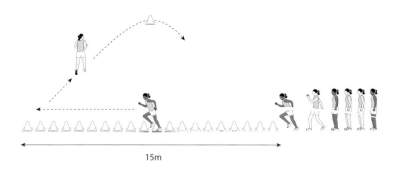

15m

Objective: To develop agility, speed, fitness and change of direction

Equipment: Cones or poles

Description: Mark out an equilateral triangle with sides 15m long, situated 3m apart. On one side of the triangle additional cones should be spaced approximately every 0.75m, with the other two sides having a cone at each end to mark the 15m distance. Get the children into teams of 8 – although you can have as many as 12 in each team. Line them up on the side of the triangle with the evenly spaced multiple cones. Each young person in the team starts off at intervals on your command, and they slalom in and out of the cones, and then run the other sides of the triangle back to the start position as quickly as they can. Change the direction of the run, alternating from starting on the left and right corners.

Coaching points: The children should ensure that they skip through the cones with quick feet.

Variation: Lay out two triangles and have teams of equal numbers. Run as a relay race with the children touching hands to change over.

Do: Ten sets of runs, five starting from a left corner and five from a right corner.

Intensity: High

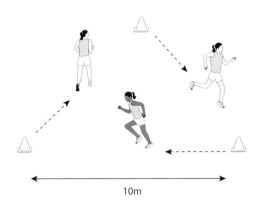

10m

Objective: To develop agility, speed, fitness and change of direction

Equipment: Cones or poles

Description: Mark out two equilateral triangles. Put the children into teams of three. The three children start on a cone and attempt to catch the player in front of them. The first three rest while the next three work. You can involve 9–12 children in each group which will extend the recovery time.

Coaching points: The children should skip round the cones with quick feet.

Variation: Change the direction of the run, alternating the side from which the drill is started or you could set up two or more triangles with mirroring layouts and swap the teams over.

Do: Two sets of five runs from each side.

Intensity: High

drill 83 '5-5-5 and run'

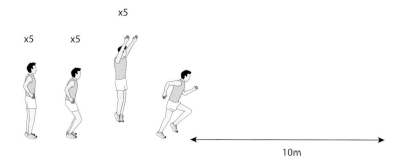

x5   x5   x5

10m

Objective: To develop power and speed

Description: The children stand with their hands on their hips. They do five slow squats, five fast squats, five double-footed jumps for height, land from the last jump and sprint 10 metres.

Coaching points: The children should run using their arms, but they must complete all the squat variants with their hands on their hips.

Do: Four sets with 90 seconds rest between sets and a walk back recovery between repetitions.

Intensity: High

drill 84 piggy-back squats

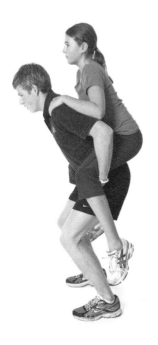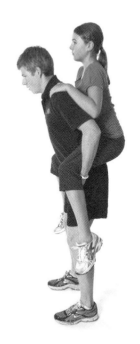

Objective: To develop strength

Description: Pair the children by height and weight. On your command 'A' jumps onto the back of 'B' and 'B' does 10 slow half squats. On completion the children change over.

Coaching points: The children must work together. They should squat down so their thighs are near parallel to the ground position. It must be stressed that the squats need to be performed slowly and with control – it is not a race.

Do: Three sets of 10 reps with 30 seconds rest between sets, and the children alternating positions.

Intensity: Medium

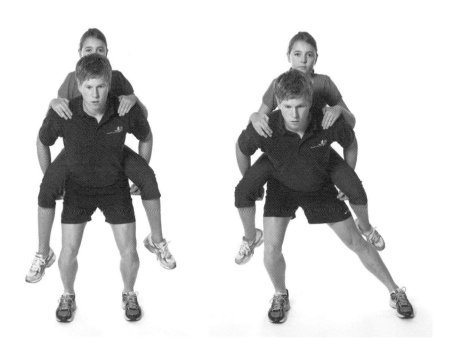

Objective: To develop strength and team work.

Description: Pair players by height and weight. On your command 'A' jumps onto the back of 'B' and 'B' and starts walking sideways for 5m. They then walk back and, at the start position, change over.

Coaching points: The children must work together. They should walk slowly and with control – it is not a race.

Do: Three sets of 5 reps with 30 seconds rest between sets, and children alternating positions and the direction of the walk.

Intensity: Medium

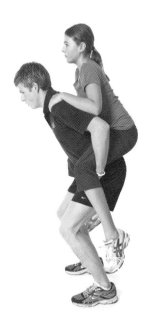 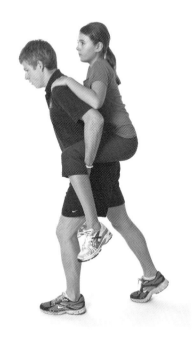

Objective: To develop strength and team work

Description: The drill is performed in the same way as drill 84, except that after completing the 10 squats, 'B' walks 10m. At the end of the walk, players should reverse roles and the drill is repeated with the pair returning to the start position.

Coaching points: The walk should be completed slowly – it is not a race. You may wish to discard the 10 squats after the piggy-back has been formed when first teaching this drill.

Do: Five walks each with 60 seconds rest in between sets.

Intensity: High

high-five

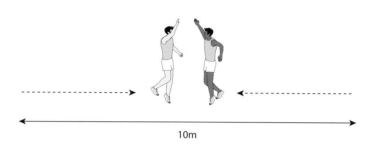

10m

Objective: To develop power, strength and coordination

Description: Working in pairs, the children line up 10m apart facing each other. On your command the children run to their partner and jump to do a high-five with their right hand. They then walk back to their start positions.

Coaching points: The players must work together to time their jumps.

Do: Five high-fives to the right and five to the left taking 20 seconds rest between jumps.

Intensity: Medium

drill 88 ball pick up

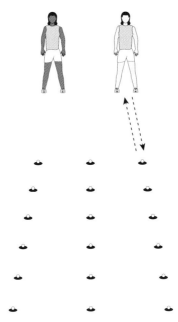

Objective: To develop speed, acceleration and fitness

Equipment: Six marker spots, six tennis balls

Description: Space the marker spots in lines of three, one metre apart and place a tennis ball on each. The children work in pairs. One player starts off 4m back from the first right hand marker spot and in line with it. Mark this position with a cone. On your command,they run to the first marker spot in the first line on the right and pick the ball up with their right hand. They turn and sprint back to the start position where they put the ball down (you could use a bin or a basket). They turn again and sprint back to the next marker spot in the first line and return with the ball to the start position, using their right hand to pick it up. The drill is continued until all the balls have been collected.

The other player returns the balls to the marker spots and then gets ready for their turn. After this the first player (having recovered) re-positions the balls and goes again, this time from the left hand side of the grid and using their left hand to grab the balls from the marker spots. When they have finished, their partner re-positions the balls and gets ready to have their turn from the left.

Coaching points: The children should pace themselves as the constant stop, start, turning and sprinting is tiring. It's best to stay low while performing the drill.

Variation: Add another row of marker spots and cones or time the drill.

Do: One rep from each side of the grid.

Intensity: High

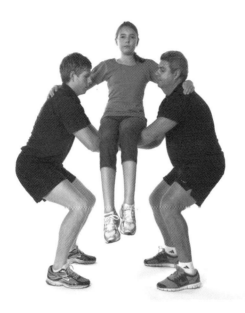

Objective: To develop team work and strength

Equipment: Cones

Description: Set up an area 10m long with cones. Get the children into teams of three. On your command, two of the children form a 'chair' by linking arms and the third player jumps onto the chair. The children then race to the 10m line where they change over, so that a different person is carried. They then run back to the start, and change again so that the last player is carried.

Coaching points: Ensure the children are of similar height and weight and are able to lift each other.

Do: Three runs per team.

Intensity: High

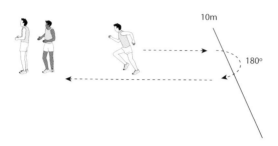

Objective: To develop acceleration, agility and team work

Equipment: Cones

Description: Set up an area of 10 metres long with cones. Get the children into teams of three. On your command, the first player runs backwards to the 10 metre line, turns through 180 degrees and runs backwards to their team mates. When they pass the line, the next person sets off. The drill is completed when the third member of the team has had their turn.

Coaching points: Children should run on the balls of their feet, and coordinate their arms with their legs (see drill 14). Ensure that there is sufficient space between the teams and that that there are no trip hazards.

Do: Three runs per team.

Intensity: Medium

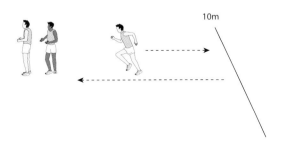

10m

Objective: To develop acceleration, agility and team work

Equipment: Cones

Description: Set up an area 10m long with cones. Get the children into teams of three. On your command, the first player runs backwards to the 10m line, then runs forwards towards the rest of the team. When they pass the next person in line, that player sets off. The drill is completed when the third runner has had their turn.

Coaching points: The children should run on the balls of their feet, and coordinate their arms with their legs (see drill 14). Ensure that there is sufficient space between the teams and that that there are no trip hazards.

Do: Three runs per team.

Intensity: High

dolphins v sharks

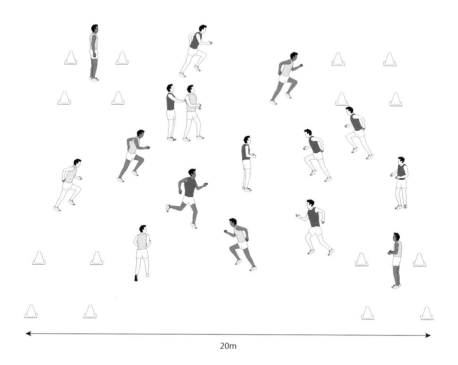

20m

Objective: To develop, fitness and acceleration

Equipment: Cones

Description: With cones, mark an area 20m square and in each corner create another 1m square. Four 'sharks' patrol the area between the squares while two 'dolphins' hide in each of the squares. On your command, the dolphins attempt to run between each of the small squares while the sharks try and catch them. When a dolphin is caught they have to leave the game by stepping into the small squares. To get caught, sharks have to touch the dolphins by placing one hand on their back. The dolphins can free the other dolphins by stepping into the small squares.

Coaching points: Encourage light and fast movements made on the balls of the feet. Children should keep their heads up to see where they are going.

Do: Four games.

Intensity: High

single leg hop relay

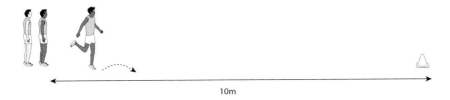

10m

Objective: To develop fitness and agility, coordination and strength

Equipment: Cones

Description: Get the children into teams of five, lined up one behind the other and at least a metre apart. Place cones 10m in front of the teams. The children start hopping on their left leg and hop to the cone in front of them, where they turn round, change legs and hop back. The next player starts when their hand has been touched by their incoming team mate.

Coaching points: Hops should be light and ground contacts quick. The children should keep their head and chest up throughout.

Do: Four runs with 60 seconds rest between.

Intensity: High

drill 94 knee tapping

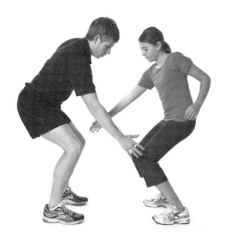 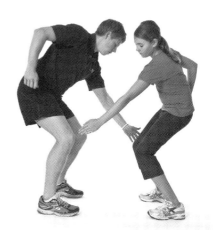

Objective: To develop fitness and agility

Description: Working in pairs, the children bend their knees to get into a crouched position. They try to tap their partner on the knee while at the same time avoiding being tapped on their own knee.

Coaching points: The children should try and tap their partner five times and whoever achieves this first is the winner. Players should be on their toes and moving all the time while remaining in the crouched position. There should be no hard hitting.

Do: Four sets of five taps, or time for 90 seconds, whichever comes first. Leave 60 seconds rest between games.

Intensity: Medium

drill 95 bean-bag steal

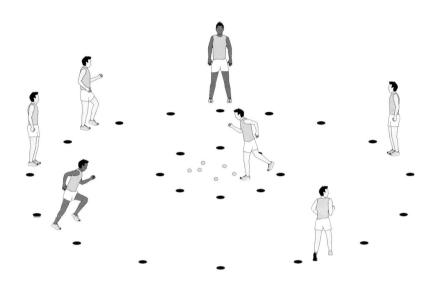

Objective: To develop agility, speed and acceleration

Equipment: Marker spots, bean-bags, whistle

Description: Using marker spots, mark out a large circle with a smaller one inside. No more than 6–8 children should be stationed around the outside of the large circle. One player (the catcher) 'defends' the inner circle, which contains the same number of bean-bags as there are children in the outer circle. The objective of the game is for the children to run slowly around the outside of the circle then, in response to your whistle, run into the inner circle and grab one of the bean-bags. Once they have moved inside the outer circle perimeter they cannot run back. If they are successful in grabbing a bean-bag, they run out of the circle and sit down. The defender has to stop them by tagging them – and those tagged must leave the game. The game is finished when all the bean-bags have been taken from the centre circle, or when all those going for the bean-bags have been tagged, or if a designated time limit is passed.

Coaching points: Encourage players to be light on their feet and to look where they are going. They should make quick changes of direction to 'trick' the catcher.

Do: Two to four repetitions. Games can be limited to 2 minutes.

Intensity: High

drill 96 bulldog

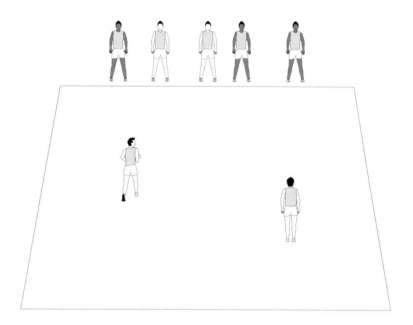

Objective: To develop speed, agility and acceleration

Equipment: Marker spots, indoor or outdoor dry surface

Description: Mark a grid approximately 20m x 10m (the width will depend on the number of children in your session). Line the children up at one end of the grid and position one or two, the 'bulldogs', in the centre. The children at the end have to get across to the other side without being tagged. If they are, they have to join the others in the centre of the grid. The game continues until all the players in the grid have been tagged. Tags are made by touching the player's back with the palm of one hand.

Coaching points: Movements must be dynamic and made from the balls of the feet. Children must keep their heads up so they can see where they are going!

Variations: Scarves can be tucked into the back of children's shorts to make tails and the bulldog has to grab these to tag the player.

Do: Two games.

Intensity: Medium

obstacle courses

Children love a challenge and obstacle courses can be a great way to develop virtually all aspects of fitness – agility, strength, speed, reaction, body awareness and coordination – all the elements of fitness which we have described in earlier sections.

Courses can be made using basic equipment, such as hoops, marker spots and cones. They can be created indoors or out and can be done individually or on a team basis as relay races. We have provided you with some examples in this section. Use your imagination and the equipment you have available to create your own variations.

Obstacle courses could form a class or a workout in their own right. You would start by teaching the individual components and their skill requirements, before letting the children complete the whole course in one go using all the skills.

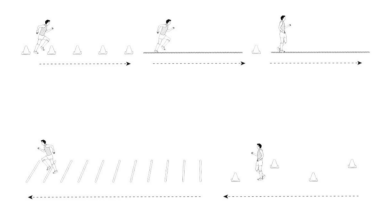

Objective: To develop all round agility and fitness

Equipment: Cones, marker spots, canes/brightly coloured tape, whistle and stop-watch

Description: Set up the obstacle course as in the diagram. Walk the young people through the course before you start, explaining all the different elements. If you have enough people in your group, you could create teams and record the time each team takes to complete the course. This would add a competitive element. Change-overs must be monitored and these should be made with the incoming runner touching the outstretched hand, held to the side of the body, of the next person.

Coaching points: Although this drill is great fun, you should still take time to coach the techniques of the specific sections of the obstacle course. All movements should be made quickly and dynamically and usually from the balls of the feet.

Do: Three times.

Intensity: High

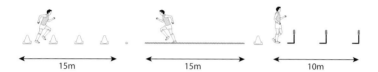

15m   15m   10m

Equipment: Cones, bean-bags, mini hurdles

Description: This uses relatively little equipment and can therefore be set up easily and quickly. Put the children into teams and line them up behind identical obstacle courses. In turn, the children slalom in and out of the cones, stop, pick up one of a number of bean-bags, put it on their head and walk or run 15m to put the bean-bag down by the cone. If the bean-bag falls off their head then they have to pick it up and return to the bean-bag part of the course. They then hurdle the mini-hurdles, run round the cone and sprint back to the start to hand over to the next person in their team.

Coaching points: As with drill 97, take time to coach the techniques for specific sections of the obstacle course and look back on the drills dealing with agility.

Do: Three times.

Intensity: High

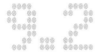

relay races

Many drills can be performed as relay races, but here are some specific examples. They are great fun and, like the games and obstacle courses, make a great way to end a session. They can incorporate many of the drills or elements of the drills which we have described in previous sections.

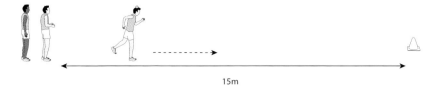

15m

Objective: To develop fitness, balance and body awareness

Equipment: Bean-bags, cones

Description: Line the children up one behind the other in teams. Position a cone 15m in front of each team. On your command, the first runner puts a bean-bag on their head and runs to and around the cone in front of them, and back to the next runner in their team. The bean-bag is handed over and the next runner completes the course with the bean-bag on their head. The relay is finished when the last runner returns and the team sits on the ground in a straight line. If the bean-bag falls to the floor during the race the runner must pick it up, return to the start and run their leg again.

Coaching points: Stress the need for controlled speed and an upright posture – hands cannot be used to re-balance the bean-bags once running.

Do: Four races.

Intensity: Medium

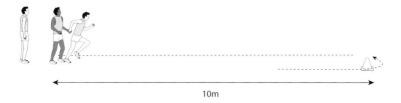

10m

Objective: To develop, speed, agility and team work

Equipment: Cones

Description: Ask the children to line up, one behind the other, in teams of three. Position a cone 15m in front of each team. On your command the first runner runs to the cone, around it and back to their team. They take the hand of the second runner and the two of them run together around the cone and back. They grab the third runner by the hand and the three of them set off again. The race is completed when the trio races back to the start line, and sits on the floor in a straight line.

Coaching points: Make sure the runners run together and don't tug too hard on each other (let them know that if the chain breaks they have to run that leg again). Each member of the team should have a go as the first, second and third runner so that they all put in the same amount of effort (the person who runs first has to do the most running).

Do: Three races so that each child runs the same distance.

Intensity: High

shuttle relay

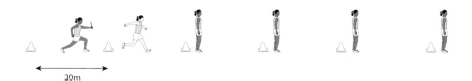

20m

Equipment: Relay batons, cones

Description: Place six cones in a straight line 20 m apart (you will need to do this exercise outside unless you have a big indoor hall). One member of each team stands behind each cone facing forward. The starting runner holds a relay baton. On your command they sprint to the next cone and hand the baton over to the person in front of them and remain on that person's cone. This continues until they get to the last cone. The last runner turns and runs all the way back to the beginning of the line to find the next runner. The baton should be held upright and the outgoing child should have their right hand up ready to collect it. The race is finished when all team members have returned to their original starting position.

Coaching points: This is simply a test of speed, but encourage the children to drive their arms backwards and forwards in time with their legs, and to keep their heads up.

Do: Three times

Variation: Increase the number of runs made by each child or increase the distance run each time.

Intensity: High